Acidophilus

by DEANNE TENNEY

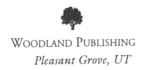

WOODLAND PUBLISHING
Pleasant Grove, UT

Contents

Acidophilus

INTRODUCTION

Nutritional supplements are increasing in popularity. As more individuals become aware of the their nutritional deficiencies, natural approaches to replenishing the body are being sought. The digestive system has often been overlooked as a factor in overall body health. If food and supplements are not absorbed and assimilated, the nutrients may not reach the bloodstream to nourish the entire body. Acidophilus is a supplement found in the body necessary for digestion, assimilation and in protecting the health of the intestinal tract.

Each body has its own ecosystem. Trillions of microorganisms live inside everyone. These microorganisms coexist within the body and are necessary for health and vitality. The beneficial bacteria help in extracting nutrients and protecting the body from detrimental factors. The intestinal microflora perform many essential functions , and have the ability of changing according to environmental and dietary changes.[1]

Bacteria has a negative connotation because most individuals associate bacteria with infections and illness. Intestinal bacteria are necessary for body health and in the prevention of disease. In recent years different strains of drug resistant bacteria have emerged due to an overuse and misuse of antibiotics. Most often the bacteria can coexist without causing harm. And there are certain bacterias which are necessary for a healthy body that actually help to keep the negative bacteria under control. Lactobacillus acidophilus is one bacteria essential in maintaining a healthy intestinal flora.

Acidophilus is the primary friendly bacteria found in the intestinal tract and vagina. They help to protect the body from an invasion of candida and other germs that invade and live in the body. Lactobacillus acidophilus helps by adhering to the intestinal wall and preventing disease causing bacteria from taking hold. They cover the lining of the intestines leaving no space for detrimental organisms to reside. When the good bacteria are compromised, space is made for the invading organisms to take hold. They also help by eating all the food reserves and starving out the bad bacteria and allowing them to pass through without taking up residence. Acidophilus is also responsible for producing acetic acids which lower the natural pH in the intestines which discourages the growth of the other bacteria which flourish in a more acidic environment. Lactobacillus acidophilus, along with other beneficial bacteria, produces an antibiotic like substance that works against other bacteria, viruses, protozoa and fungi.[2] They work to protect the body from invaders.

Lactobacillus acidophilus is the most prevalent form of beneficial bacteria found in the small intestine. It is estimated that a healthy colon should contain at least 85 percent lactobacillus and 15 percent coliform bacteria.[3] Most individuals are lacking in the necessary levels of Lactobacillus which contributes to digestive disorders such as gas, bloating, constipation, malabsorption of nutrients, and heartburn.

Acidophilus bacteria also help by detoxifying some harmful substances in the gastrointestinal tract. They also aid in the digestion of proteins which is essential for the production of essential enzymes made in the body. Lactobacillus acidophilus also helps to manufacture B vitamins such as B1, B2, B3, B12 and folic acid.

The intestinal flora can be affected by various elements. The overuse of antibiotics, oral contraceptives, excessive sugar consumption, aspirin, antihistamines, cortisone, prednisone, coffee and stress can all contribute to an imbalance in the bacterial flora of the gastrointestinal tract. When the friendly bacteria are outnumbered, detrimental substances may not be excreted from the body leading to unhealthy conditions. We come into contact with harmful bacteria on a daily basis. When Lactobacillus acidophilus is flourishing in the digestive tract, we have an added protection from infection and disease.

Antibiotics: Friend or Foe?

There is no doubt that antibiotics have saved numerous lives since their development. But many health care providers in the past have seen them as a panacea for all ailments including viral infections that are not affected by antibiotic therapy. They have been overused and with disastrous results. Antibiotics are used to help the body in fighting infection, but unfortunately, they also may encourage recurrent infections caused by a destruction of the good as well as the bad bacteria lowering the immune function and leading to a dependence on antibiotics. Because of an overuse and misuse of antibiotics, some forms of bacteria are now resistant to them. Diseases which were aided with antibiotic therapy are now resistant to the treatment. Antibiotics are sometimes prescribed by physicians even when they are not appropriate.[4]

Medical professionals almost felt guilty a few years ago when not prescribing some form of antibiotic when patients visited the office. After all, what good is a doctor if the patient does not leave with a cure. Fortunately, most doctors now know the detrimental affects that can follow excessive and inappropriate use of antibiotics. Most doctors now will be honest and up front with their patients when there is not a cure-all answer to their problem. An investigative reporter a few years ago visited a number of physicians around the country asking for antibiotics. It was interesting to note that almost all of the physicians agreed to prescribing antibiotics upon the patients request even when it wasn't warranted. In being confronted after, most replied that they had to do what the patient asked in order to keep their practice flourishing. No wonder antibiotic overuse has resulted in drug-resistant strains of bacteria.

The negative affects of antibiotics are well known. Antibiotics interfere with the growth of bacteria, both good and bad. But they are crafty creatures and have the ability of changing their chemistry and genes to avoid destruction by antibiotics. They want to survive and thrive. They grow at a very rapid rate allowing for a whole generation of drug resistant strains to develop in just a relatively short period of time. Alexander Fleming, who discovered penicillin, warned of the problem that could occur with resistant strains if antibiotics were overused.[5] The weaker bacteria may be killed while the stronger endure. This causes the strong, resistant bacteria to invade and take hold in the body.

Mitchell L. Cohen, a researcher with the National Center for Infectious Diseases at the Centers for Disease Control, issued this warning about antibiotics in 1992: "Unless currently effective antimicrobial agents can be successfully preserved and the transmission of drug-resistant organisms curtailed, the post-antimicrobial era may be rapidly approaching in which infectious disease ward housing untreatable conditions will again be seen." Patients, doctors, scientists and public health officials must all play their part in finding ways to reduce reliance upon antibiotics.[6]

Lactobacillus acidophilus is one of the most essential bacteria found in the intestinal tract. It helps to keep the disease causing organisms under control. Antibiotics can reduce the quantities of good and bad bacteria often allowing negative organisms to flourish. Broad spectrum antibiotics are the worst offenders often making way for an overgrowth of yeast which can affect the entire body. The broad spectrum antibiotics work just as they are called, broadly throughout the body, to kill just about all the bacteria around. If an antibiotic is warranted, the most specific type for the condition should be tried first in order to protect as much of the normal intestinal flora as possible.

When taking antibiotics, Lactobacillus acidophilus can be taken by mouth to help restore normal intestinal flora. Acidophilus will not interfere with the effectiveness of the antibiotics but protect and aid in the healing process. Antibiotic use should be minimized; used only when essential to health and survival. The beneficial bacteria are the first to be destroyed from the antibiotic therapy. Lactobacillus acidophilus can also help to fight the bad bacteria and organisms that invade the body.

Acidophilus: Nature's Antibiotic

Lactobacillus acidophilus has been found to contain antibiotic properties. According to Dr. Khem Shahani, a professor of food science at the University of Nebraska, milk fermented by Lactobacillus acidophilus contains an antibiotic he calls "acidophilin." It is a powerful antibiotic with similar abilities as penicillin, streptomycin and terramycin. He actually believes that it is more powerful than the antibiotics mentioned.[7]

Detrimental bacteria invade our bodies on a daily basis. Supplementing with either yogurt containing live cultures or a freeze dried capsule may be necessary to protect the body. Lactobacillus acidophilus can protect the digestive system from microorganisms causing infection and disease. It is a supplement that can help protect the body and work as "nature's antibiotic."

YOGURT

Plain yogurt is basically a combination of milk and Lactobacillus acidophilus, the friendly bacteria. This is the bacteria that produces lactase which aids in the process of curdling the milk and giving yogurt its tart flavor. Yogurt containing live cultures of Lactobacillus acidophilus have been found effective in treating vaginal yeast infections, infant diarrhea, food poisoning, and in preventing flu infections.[8]

Yogurt must contain the live, active cultures of Lactobacillus acidophilus to be beneficial. The intestinal flora can be disrupted by conditions such as antibiotic therapy, stress, a poor diet, excess sugar consumption, and oral contraceptives. This friendly bacteria is not destroyed by the acidic gastric juices in the stomach and protects the body by adhering to the intestinal wall. Yogurt is a great way to add the beneficial bacteria often needed in the body. Some physicians recommend plain yogurt to patients undergoing antibiotic therapy to counteract the negative effects of the antibiotic.

Many of the commercial brands of yogurt found in the neighborhood grocery store do not contain live, active cultures. Check carefully to assure the best quality available. Most health food stores have specialty brands with live cultures.

Candida Yeast Infections

Many women are plagued with a constant battle with yeast infections. It is one of the most common reasons women visit a physician. It can be a very annoying condition often causing pain and discomfort. Candida albicans is commonly found on the skin, mouth, digestive tract and the vagina. Candida is a fungus found in the body all the time. Normally it does not pose a threat because the numbers are kept under control by the beneficial bacteria (acidophilus). When an imbalance of the bacteria occurs, the candida can flourish sometimes leading to serious conditions.

Antibiotic therapy, oral contraceptives, douching, and female hygiene sprays can all destroy the beneficial bacteria needed in the body and allow the candida to proliferate. Antibiotics are often used to treat yeast infections when they may be the initial culprit. Broad spectrum antibiotics can destroy the beneficial bacteria in the vagina allowing the yeast to grown. Using antibiotics to treat the condition can destroy the remaining good bacteria leading to a dependency on antibiotic treatment. Pregnancy can also cause disturbances in the intestinal flora.[9] Whenever a disturbance in the bacterial flora occurs, it is important to take measures to reestablish the normal balance of friendly bacteria.

One study found that women who consumed one cup daily of yogurt with the live Lactobacillus acidophilus cultures had a reduction in candida infections. The acidophilus does not kill the candida but helps to encourage an environment more suitable for the the beneficial bacteria to live and grow.[10] Eileen Hilton M.D., a specialist at the Long Island Jewish Medical Center in New York, followed 11 women with chronic yeast infections. They ate one cup daily of yogurt rich in live Lactobacillus acidophilus. During the last six months of the study, the women averaged only one yeast infection.[11]

Another study done by Alexander Neri, M.D. a the Beilinson Medical Center in Israel followed 32 women with bacterial vaginosis. They were asked to apply yogurt with Lactobacillus acidophilus twice a day for two weeks. Then they were told to skip a week and start again. After two days of treatment, all the women had recovered. All but four remained free of symptoms for two months.[12]

Other studies have also confirmed the benefits of Lactobacillus acidophilus in treating Candida albicans. Many beneficial results have been found using this natural form of treatment that enhances the body and encourages the growth of helpful bacteria rather than destroying all bacteria.

CHOLESTEROL LEVELS

High cholesterol levels have been linked to many serious conditions such as heart disease and cancer. Acidophilus seems promising in helping to lower cholesterol levels. It may work by converting cholesterol to coprostanol which is not absorbed in the body; thus working to lower overall body cholesterol levels.[13]

Some research has found that Lactobacillus acidophilus may help to lower blood cholesterol levels.[14] Blood cholesterol levels of 54 volunteers were monitored. Volunteers were given either milk or yogurt containing Lactobacillus acidophilus. After one week, the individuals given the yogurt had lowered their cholesterol levels by five to ten percent.[15]

A study involving pigs also found beneficial effects in lowering cholesterol using Lactobacillus acidophilus. Pigs were fed pure crystalline cholesterol. One group received acidophilus in their diet while another was not. The animals receiving the acidophilus showed lower gains in serum cholesterol levels.[16]

Lactose Intolerance

Lactose intolerance is a common condition. It occurs as the body is not able to digest the milk sugar found in dairy products. Symptoms can include stomach cramps, gas, diarrhea, indigestion and general stomach discomfort. Some individuals have a difficult time digestive and assimilating milk products.

Acidophilus has been added to some commercial brands of milk products to aid in digestion. The addition of Lactobacillus acidophilus has been found to help improve lactose absorption and reduce the problems of some people with lactose intolerance. The acidophilus contains an enzyme that may be missing in individuals with lactose intolerance. This enzyme is responsible for changing the lactose to lactic acid. One study found that the addition of acidophilus to low fat milk improved the lactose absorption by four times in lactose sensitive individuals. The results were better over a week period and lasted for a week after the discontinuation of the acidophilus milk.[17]

CANCER

The area which encompasses the digestive tract is large which leads to a high degree of exposure to harmful substances that enter the body. Evidence seems to point to the possibility of Lactobacillus acidophilus in the prevention of cancer, mainly colon cancer. A Boston scientist found that acidophilus cultures can help by suppressing the activity in the colon that can allow for the conversion of harmful substances into carcinogens.[18] The acidophilus produces metabolites that help inhibit the growth of bacteria that can produce carcinogens.

Yogurt with active cultures has been found to help the growth of friendly bacteria and suppress the growth of cancer cells. A Polish study found that bowel cancer patients fed one quart of yogurt a day for two months resulted in cancer reduction in ten of those patients.[19]

The effects of the acidophilus seem to be more pronounced in individuals who eat meat. When a supplement was given to vegetarians, there was only a small decrease in enzymes known to turn substances into carcinogens. But in the group who eat meat there was a two to four fold decrease in the enzymes. The change occurred over a period of one to two weeks and continued as long as the Lactobacillus acidophilus supplements were given.[20]

One French study found that women who ate diets high in cheese and dairy fat had a higher risk of breast cancer. Those who ate yogurt in their diets on a regular basis had the lowest risk for breast cancer.[21]

Immune System Enhancer

Intestinal bacteria are important in preventing disease. Researchers at the Institute for Medicine, Microbiology and Hygiene at the University of Cologne in France, have been studying the benefits of bacteria in the intestinal tract. They have found that intestinal bacteria, such as L. acidophilus, produce peptides, which are made from amino acids, and help to increase the immunity in the body.[22] One study done used antibiotics to destroy the beneficial bacteria and lower immunity. The peptides were introduced and immunity was improved.[23]

"Animal experiments have found that common strains of L. acidophilus, L. casei, L. bulgaricus and S. thermophilus (found in yogurt products) enhance the bacteria-eating ability of white blood cells. In a remarkable human study, Georges M. Halpern, M.D., of the University of California, Davis, reported that "live-culture" yogurt dramatically boosted the body's production of immune-stimulating interferon."[24]

Constipation

Constipation can occur for many reasons. Lactobacillus acidophilus has been found to help.

Regular bowel function can help protect the body from possible carcinogenic activity. The faster matter moves through the bowels, the less chance of healthy cells being attacked.

A study reported in the Journal of the American Medical Association involved 194 hospitalized individuals with constipation problems. The average age of the volunteers was 72 years and none of them were being hospitalized for serious illnesses. They were given a daily dose of Lactobacillus acidophilus in a yogurt-prune whip dessert. Over 95 percent of the patients soon were off laxatives as long as they continued eating the nightly dessert.[25]

DIARRHEA

Not only is acidophilus helpful in cases of constipation but it also helps with diarrhea. Diarrhea can occur with a disturbance of the intestinal bacterial flora. Lactose intolerance can also lead to diarrhea. Eating yogurt with active acidophilus cultures or a supplement can help restore the normal flora and help diarrhea.

A study done by Heikki Vapatalo, M.D., involved 16 healthy men taking erythromycin, which is an antibiotic known to cause diarrhea. One group was given two cups daily of yogurt with live cultures and the other pasteurized yogurt. The group with the live cultures recovered in two days from diarrhea while the other took eight days to show improvement.[26]

Other studies have found beneficial results in treating traveler's diarrhea with acidophilus. Many individuals routinely take L. acidophilus supplements when traveling out of the country because of the possibility of contaminated food and water.

BABIES AND ACIDOPHILUS

Babies first come into contact with L. acidophilus as they pass through the vagina during the birth process. Babies born by Cesarean section often have a harder time adjusting a healthy flora in their intestinal tracts. Breast fed babies receive acidophilus through colostrum in the mother's milk.[27]

A group of infants were given yogurt with active cultures after antibiotic treatment. The stools of the infants were high in disease causing bacteria after the antibiotics. After three weeks of the yogurt treatment, their intestinal flora was healthy.[28]

Other Beneficial Bacteria

LACTOBACILLUS BULGARICUS

This is another of the beneficial bacteria sometimes found in the intestinal tract. Though not always found in the body, it helps to produce lactic acid and has some antibiotic activity beneficial to health.[29] Studies have found that Lactobacillus bulgaricus can help to increase immune function aiding in healing and the prevention of infections.[30]

LACTOBACILLUS CASEI SSP. RHAMNOSUS

This is a beneficial bacteria similar to acidophilus. Some believe that because of their close similarities, they may have been confused in the past to some degree. This good bacteria grows rapidly and aid in boosting the immune response.[31]

LACTOBACILLUS BIFIDUS

This beneficial bacteria is often found in the large intestinal and vagina. It is often found in the normal intestinal flora of infants and children. For this reason, some children's supplements have been formulated containing this bacteria along with others. Breast milk has been found to contain Lactobacillus bifidus. It has also been found to help protect infants against intestinal infections, an overgrowth of candida following antibiotic therapy and in breaking down lactose for those with lactose intolerance.[32]

STREPTOCOCCUS FAECIUM

This is another beneficial component of the intestinal tract. It helps to produce large amounts of lactic acid. It reproduces rapidly, contains resistance to acidic conditions, contains antibiotic activity, aids in returning the normal flora to the intestinal tract after antibiotic therapy and is heat resistant up to 90 degrees F.

Supplements

Supplements of Lactobacillus acidophilus can be bought at health food stores. They are generally found in dried, powdered or liquid cultures. Most forms are milk based though some nondairy versions have been cultured with a carrot juice base. The capsules or liquid contain higher quantities of the acidophilus than yogurt, acidophilus milk or other milk products. All supplements should be refrigerated after opening.

The most beneficial effects from supplements of acidophilus are achieved when taken on an empty stomach when the acid level is at its lowest point. This helps the acidophilus to make its way to the intestines where it can do the most good.[33]

Conclusion

Most of the microorganisms within our bodies are not harmful. They help to control and discourage the bad bacteria from taking up residence. So it is important to encourage the growth of the beneficial bacteria to ensure health and vitality.

Lactobacillus acidophilus is an important part of the intestinal flora. It is essential to our very existence and health. Benefits will be felt if the beneficial bacteria are allowed to flourish and thrive making a less hospitable environment for the disease causing organisms to live.

Endnotes

1Chriostpher Hobbs, Foundations of Health, The Liver and Digestive Herbal, (Capitola, CA: Botanica Press, 1992), 63.

2Jack Challem, "Good Bacteria that Fight the Bad," Let's Live. (October, 1995) 55.

3James F. Balch, M.D. and Patricia A. Balch, C.N.C., Prescription For Nutritional Healing. (Garden City Park, N.Y.: Avery Publishing Group Inc., 1990), 37.

4Michael A. Schmidt, Lendon H. Smith and Keith W. Sehnert, Beyond Antibiotics, (Berkeley: North Atlantic Books, 1994), 14,15.

5Ibid., 19.

6M.L. Cohen, "Epidemiology of drug resistance: implications for a post-antimicrobial era," Science, (1992; 257) 1050-1055. cited in Michael A. Schmidt, 21.

7James F. Scheer, "Acidophilus, Nautre's Antibiotic," Better Nutrition For Today's Living, (August, 1993), 34.

8Phyllis A. Balch, C.N.C. and James F. Balch, M.D., Prescription for Cooking and Dietary Wellness. (Greenfield, Indiana: P.A.B. Publishing, Inc., 1987) 187.

9Elizabeth Somer, M.A., R.D., Nutrition For Women, The Complete Guide. (New York: Henry Holt and Company, 1993) 382,383.

10Ibid., 384.

11Michael Castleman, Nature's Cures. (Emmaus, Pennsylvania: Rodale Press, Inc., 1996), 176.

12Alexander Neri, M.D., Acta Obstetriia Gynecologica Scandinavaca. (Jan. 1993; 72) 17-19. cited in Jack Challem, Let's Live, 56.

13Hobbs, 70.

14Phyllis A. Balch, 188.

15Scheer, 37.

16Marcia Starck, The Complete Handbook of Natural Healing, (St. Paul: Llewellyn Publications, 1993), 68.

17Hobbs, 98.

18Phyllis A. Balch, 188.

19Ibid., 188.

20Hobbs, 99.

21Ibid., 188.

22Challem, 55.

23Ibid., 55

24International Journal of Immunotherapy. (1991; 7: 205-210) cited in Challem, 55.

25Scheer, 36.

26Challem, 56.

27Jack Ritchason, Vitamin and Health Encyclopedia. (Pleasant Grove, UT: Woodland Books, 1994), p 34.

28Scheer, 36.

29Hobbs, 100.

30Ibid., 66.

31 Ibid., 100
32 Ibid., 100.
33 Scheer, 37.